Ruth started work at 16 years of age, working for a utility company in North West England. It was here she met Neil and they got married in 1989. Both have a common love of travelling. They enjoy the histories and cultures of different places, the various culinary delights and the stories and myths that bring a place to life. The love of the sea is another passion and they are happiest at their 'Sanctuary by the Sea', their static caravan on Llŷn, Wales.

To my husband, your love and strength make everything bearable.

To Moe and Graham, your time and company means so much.

To all my family and friends, I thank you all.

In tears of laughter and tears of pain, you're the people who kept me sane.

Ruth Roche

KEEPING ABREAST OF THE SITUATION

AUSTIN MACAULEY PUBLISHERS™

LONDON • CAMBRIDGE • NEW YORK • SHARJAH

A CIP catalogue record for this title is available from the British Library.

ISBN 9781398408326 (Paperback)
ISBN 9781398408333 (ePub e-book)

www.austinmacauley.com

First Published (2021)
Austin Macauley Publishers Ltd
25 Canada Square
Canary Wharf
London
E14 5LQ

The Beginning

I was 48 when I received my first invitation to attend a mammogram. I was one of the selected few of that age. I had no family history of breast cancer. I knew what the test consisted of; potentially the most uncomfortable ten minutes of my life (apart from the dreaded smear which could only ever be comfortable to a prostitute with a medical fetish!!!) I attended that first flat tit test, and two weeks later received the all clear.

After breaking the ½ century big birthday, an achievement in itself, I am 51 when I receive another invitation to attend a second flat tit test. At this point in my life, my breasts are just part of my female anatomy. In hindsight, that's all they have ever been. They never took on the role of the cow's udder, providing milk to offspring, and have spent most of their time strapped up during the day and swinging about at night.

The invitation I have received is not to a mobile unit in my local medical centre car park but to a mobile unit in Salford precinct. The problem with this invitation is that it is bloody inconvenient. I am busy at work and don't have a clue where this medical caravan is located. I decide I'll wait until it's more local. At this point my husband, Neil, announces that he knows exactly where this scan unit can be found and he will come with me.

We live in Eccles, one of the districts within Salford City Council jurisdiction. Our house is a short stroll from the Trafford Centre (known by some as the 'stress centre') which we visit as a necessity rather than a luxury (and preferably never over the Christmas period). We are central to motorway links, Metrolink routes to Manchester city centre (and places further afield) and the town centres of Eccles and Salford. Despite the promises of regeneration, both these town centres are run down. Any artwork is graffiti, high-rise tower blocks dominate the skyline overlooking the precinct areas where pubs, bookmakers and pound shops outnumber the food retailers and supermarkets (whatever happened to the traditional butchers, bakers and greengrocers? They are now lost in commercialisation. They have been swept away on the tidal increase in business rates and lost to the corporate giants of Tesco, Sainsbury's etc. and their acres of convenience 'under one roof shopping').

This particular day, I find myself chauffeuring my other half to an appointment that is not his, knowing I am to be manhandled (or should I say woman-handled) by some unsympathetic nurse who will work through a conveyor belt of females to stretch, squash and manipulate each breast into any abnormal shape required.

We pull up in a pay-and-display car park on a grey overcast day. The sky blends in with the concrete tower blocks bearing down on this small square of tarmac. Intermittent patches of colour lighten up the neighbourhood, remnants left by the delinquents whose appreciation of art is a spray can and a blank wall. A gallery of abstract designs, alongside their appreciation of the English language and literature announcing that "Gaz woz 'ere".

We enter the health centre where we are directed along a maze of corridors into the car park at the back. The mobile unit reminds me of my primary school porta cabin. Frighteningly the nurse reminds me of a previous headmistress, friendly on the outside but with that underlying hard stare that ensures you will do everything she asks or instructs you to do.

This overall trip takes an hour out of my life.

The Referral

This appointment is now a distant memory. Two weeks have gone by and my normal life continues. The radio alarm clock continues to jumpstart my brain into life at approximately 6:15 every morning. It is still dark outside and it takes a monumental effort to swing my 'not so slim' frame towards the wall and my feet onto the plush bedroom carpet. My previous night's dream adventures are a memory. I was a heroine, Manchester's version of Lara Croft. That character has now gone—hidden, invisible, embedded in the warmth of that inviting pillow and the 13.5 tog duvet that was the deadly serpent I wrestled with on the banks of Manchester Ship Canal. Of course this is a dream battle I won. Now I am a mundane analyst listening to the radio presenter telling me what the temperature will be for the rest of the day. All I care about at this moment in time is that it is still dark…and I've misplaced a sock!!!

It is at this time of the year that I have that tinge of resentment towards those people who are retired. Neil retired three years ago. It was enforced through work circumstances and he was in danger of having a breakdown, however, he was fortunate enough to have pensions in place, so resigned with his head held high and his mind in a far better place.

Being younger than him, I still have a few years before my pension plan comes to fruition so, for now, I am the one getting dressed in the dark and peering round the curtains to see the cars glistening in the avenue, coated with the frost that no weather forecaster predicted. He remains oblivious, curled up in his cocoon snoring. Scientists reckon the average person (whatever an average person is) spends about 26 years sleeping. Neil is a firm believer that humans should hibernate as the bears do in the winter months. Thankfully he doesn't as I'm not sure when I would see him again.

At least I know my house remains clean and the washing and ironing is in safe hands. Certainly, the ironing will remain scorch-free for the foreseeable future.

Today the office staff's lunchtime discussion is about diets (not my strength—the practice, not the discussion). The newspapers are filled with the latest 'healthy options'—what is a fad? What is fashion? Vegetarianism, veganism, pescetarianism (apparently a diet that is mainly vegetarian but containing fish not meat, a prawn cocktail in my world).

My conclusion is that I like steak far too much to surrender my carnivorous tendencies. I also don't have the time or inclination to discuss which glass of alcohol is good or bad for me this week. This information is generally available through tabloid newspapers printing random scientific conclusions such as, "Cider is currently bad for me because there is an apple famine in West Kent." It is obviously all true!!!

I arrive home from work to the usual pile of random envelopes and flyers dropped through our letter box. I notice that should I decide to diet, I would get no assistance from the neighbourhood as half a dozen flyers that have been posted advertise everything from pizzas to kebabs to curries. I never receive one promoting salad with the jewellery box illustration of emerald green lettuce and ruby red tomatoes.

With these menus heading in the direction of the blue recycling bin along with the other irrelevant mail that isn't worth a stamp, I then notice THAT white envelope, the inconspicuous white windowed envelope with the unmistakeable NHS stamp.

Yes folks, the results are in!!! As with my last results I expect to pass my exam with flying colours, 'A' star and I shall resit in three years.

Ripping open the envelope as I would any other, I am nonchalantly strolling towards the paper bin when I read something I am not expecting. I have to do a resit next week. *'Please come for further tests.' 'This only happens to four in every 100 women.' 'Most women who attend the clinic do not have breast cancer.' 'You may be there for two to four hours.'* At this point. I recheck the address to confirm our postman hasn't chosen the wrong letterbox.

Now this is quite a shock to the system and not what I was expecting. Considering I was going to postpone the initial test, I now have to take more time out of work. Do people not realise I'm busy? I'm enjoying my life and job! I'm not ill, I don't feel ill and I have no lumps or bumps!

Neil is in the back bedroom doing the ironing and as I climb the stairs, I hear the dulcet tones of Phil Collins and Genesis singing *Jesus He knows me* reverberating off the walls and rattling the CD player. Well at this moment in time, I'm not sure Jesus knows anything about me. I show Neil the letter. He reassures me that everything will be fine and that we will go to Wythenshawe Hospital together.

There it is, in black and white. It is not something I can postpone or ignore, and I know it is one appointment that I cannot miss.

Patient, Patients or Patience

Tuesday, 9 April

One week later, we are sitting in the Nightingale Centre at Wythenshawe Hospital waiting for my 2 pm appointment. I am now people-watching and the thought process begins.

There is no way to categorise the people in that large waiting room. There is every gender, creed and colour. Couples, people on their own, people with their friends, families with children...and a couple of gentlemen. Of course, men can be at risk of getting breast cancer. I don't think it is something that is even acknowledged by some people and I don't think it is as publicised as it should be. Their man boobs (moobs) are often treated more light-heartedly by women, especially if the particular gentleman isn't a trained sportsman, gym attendee or carrying a six-pack.

I wonder what all these people are thinking. What do they know? A couple of younger ladies giggle like naughty schoolgirls whilst reading a *Hello!* magazine, probably viewing some celebrity wedding snaps, and slagging off the bridesmaids. They don't appear to have a care in the world. Another couple sit holding hands, no eye contact and no communication.

They stare straight ahead, in their own worlds, with their own thoughts. Some people are attached to their mobile phones, some playing games or on social media whilst others chat about their childcare or what is for tea.

I've been so busy analysing other people that I've not spoken to Neil for ten minutes, and the clock informs me that my appointment is five minutes late. The curiosity of the other clinical inmates turns into an analysis of my own predicament. *Am I in a predicament?* The medical professionals have summoned me and now they keep me waiting…ME!!! I do have other things to do and better places to be. Then my name is called and my stomach sinks. *What if?*

Neil sits in the waiting room. There is nothing he can do.

I'm taken through into a side room and find myself staring at the mammogram machine that seems to be dictating my life at the moment. Two nurses are in attendance and give me instructions. Although friendly and very softly spoken, it seems like a military drill. *Remove blouse, remove bra, arms up, turn sideways, meat on slab.* Well obviously that last phrase wasn't the actual instruction given to me but I did feel that this procedure was a bit inhuman at this time. I am being manhandled by two medical females…with cold hands…Why do they have cold hands???

Hooray. Despite the discomfort, the nurses tell me that the repeated mammogram has identified where the little inconvenience is hiding. The little discrepancy in my DNA causing all this fuss. Hardly anything to see, not a pimple to be felt. OK nothing major there! Great, I can get dressed now. In my plan, they can now give me an update on what happens next and Neil and I can go to the pub for a pint. That is a great idea. How wrong am I?

Not only am I still standing topless in this sparse room, we are now preparing for a medical procedure, the core biopsy. I use the term 'we' very lightly as I haven't got a clue what this entails and who does what. The words I hear inform me of the procedure. These include the words 'Ruth' 'anaesthetic' and 'slight pain'. It seems to resonate with me that it will be far more painful than they describe. I am not wrong.

Approximately one hour after enduring the 'tit torture chamber', I re-join Neil in the waiting area. Not the same woman that entered the pain chamber, I am now flat breasted, punctured and in pain but fully clothed and happy that it's over.

Now we sit and wait again. I have it in print that most women who attend an assessment clinic do NOT have breast cancer. My mind now wonders to the mundane…*what should we have for tea??? Will we actually be out of this medical centre in time for supper?* I would really appreciate a glass of cider at this moment in time.

Then my name is called. *What if?*

Couldn't Happen to Me

We are summoned into a small office by a nurse and told to take a seat and a consultant will see us shortly. She tells us his name. We haven't got a clue who he is but I remember that my mum's cousin by marriage is a doctor and has the same surname. Not a consultant and not a very relevant thought at this time. What a bizarre thought to have when you're about to find out that you're terminally ill. The door opens and a gentleman enters. There is no white coat, no stethoscope. In some *Mills & Boon* or *Catherine Cookson* novel, he would probably be the hero, tall and handsome, clean shaven with distinguished greying hair. Strange how his appearance has such an impact. In reality, any results would be the same whether it be Dr Kildare or Doc from the *Seven Dwarves*. A nurse follows behind like a faithful servant. Neil holds my hand. We've never been the world's greatest romantics, but this seems the most natural thing to do. The gentleman introduces himself as my consultant and introduces his colleague as my Macmillan nurse! I am no longer in my busy 'all is well with the world' life, I'm now in an 'okay, that's nice to know' moment. Then I hear THOSE words. "Your test results show you have stage one breast cancer."

That same recurring thought. *I don't feel ill. I have no lumps and bumps, apart from the natural ones* (note to self: need to lose weight).

What happens next can now only be explained as a clip from a black and white film; the world suddenly slows down and the room is void of any colour it has (which is minimal in this white clinical environment). The consultant's lips are moving but all I hear is a background drone as if his batteries are running down. Everyone is staring at me. The consultant, the nurse, my husband.

Whoa, hold the front page. Who are you talking to? Who else is in the room? ME? No? Seriously? I see tears in my husband's eyes, and then it hits me. That moment when you are emotionally looking down a tunnel and a train is thundering towards you and you can't move off the track.

The shock of that hypothetical train brings me back into the real world and real time. The consultant begins to explain what has happened and what will happen.

Apparently it's the best cancer I can have, easily treatable and a great recovery rate. How can I have breast cancer? I don't feel ill. I'm shown a diagram, a medical Picasso. The cell cluster is small, not terminal and not an emergency. I know my mother-in-law had a mastectomy operation years ago and spent her time in the ward counselling others. This result could be worse…I think! The diary comes out and like an efficient booking agent, an appointment is made for me to have surgery on Tuesday, 21 May.

Do I have any questions??? I have plenty, I just can't think of them.

Then I realise the significance of the date. Not the severity of the situation but the fact that we are going to Pisa and

Florence on holiday. We have not booked the holiday as a package, so I need to cancel the flights and contact the two hotels. Do I cancel or postpone? My life is now full of unanswered questions. In that brief sentence, my life has changed. My plans need to change. I'm not sure if my life is on hold or in freefall.

No sooner has Neil released me from the bear hug that has enveloped me for the last few minutes than then I hear that reassuring voice that tells us we can go on holiday, that nothing drastic will happen before then. "Enjoy yourselves, have a fabulous holiday, we'll see you the day after your return, on the 22 May."

Dealing

So here we are, sitting in the car wondering what has just happened. After 29 years of marriage, we don't know how to talk to each other. Do I tell people? Do they have to know? How do I tell them? What do I say? Do I tell family? I am driving out of the car park when our neighbour and close friend Moe (Maureen) rings to see how I got on. "Not as well as I hoped" is my reply. Response is: "We'll see you in the pub for a drink when you get home." This brief conversation makes my mind up, I can't hide this.

Within three hours of leaving the hospital, we are sitting in our local pub with Moe and her partner Graham telling them that I have stage one breast cancer. In hindsight, it is a surreal chat. I announce it as matter of fact. A badge of honour. It is the only way I can deal with it. The reactions are what could be classed as typical for the sex of the individual. Moe announces that she could cry, but 'puts the lid back on that bottle' as soon as it's been said. Stiff upper lip and blink a lot to disperse the tears from rolling down her cheeks. Graham gives the stoic male matter-of-fact response that it could only be good as it had been found early. Neil agrees. (Note to self: Remember generally man deals with man regarding emotion—caveman philosophy/alpha male.) The positivity is overwhelming but there is still nothing I can do to change anything.

The following day, my reality becomes normality. I return to work and tell my colleagues. The girls hold back tears and the lads are lads; strong, no emotion (caveman/alpha male response), a hug and "you'll be fine". I email my regional boss asking to see her when she is in the office. Within the hour, I am in her office. I promise myself I won't cry. Her sister-in-law had died of cancer. She was a lot younger than me, leaving a young family behind. I sit in her office, she sits next to me, and I feel tears well up. I can't look at her but stare straight through the window at the Barton High Level Bridge and tell her. She grabs some tissues and cries. My normality continues.

Nothing has changed in my work-life balance. The work continues. The same random chatter and banter. Meeting friends in the pub after work to discuss today's worldly events, gossip…and the success of the pub pool team. Yet something has changed. My thought patterns. Although I am in company, I feel like I am on the outside looking in.

I tell my close friends and neighbours. Paul and Sandra. This couple next-door have probably just been through the worst 12 months when their daughter Laura was diagnosed with cancer. A young girl who is married with two young children. She had chemotherapy, the hair loss and the pain and is now in remission. I feel the severity of my illness doesn't compare, but there are no comparisons with any form of cancer.

I need to tell my father and brother. It would be so much easier for them to remain ignorant to this until after the event. Unfortunately, I cannot go through these forthcoming medical procedures, especially any operations, with them not knowing.

Apart from their initial shock this is accepted as an inconvenience and something that will be resolved.

I receive great support, get-well cards, gifts, flowers. Again this feels bizarre. I don't feel ill. In my mind, the more people who know, the better for me. Not for sympathy but to avoid the rumour mill signing me off, kicking the proverbial bucket and putting me in an undertaker's box before my time.

A letter arrives confirming my breast abnormality requires surgery and I need to attend the Nightingale Centre on 8 May for a pre-op and a magseed (magnetic seed) to be implanted to assist in surgery. Now it's confirmed in black and white, but it's still three weeks away!!!

Easter

It is Easter weekend and ten days since the diagnosis. We are lucky to have a static caravan in Wales. We call her Vanerie and she is our 'Sanctuary by the Sea'. An investment when my mother-in-law passed away. Vanerie has two bedrooms with all mod cons (a mains gas supply and central heating—no calor gas bottles required). She has front decking so we can watch the waves break on 'Butlin's point' across the bay and a flagged drive and patio where our BBQ will take pride of place in the sunnier months. The beds are made and the wardrobes and drawers are crammed with clothing for every season and every eventuality.

My husband spent all his school holidays on this site, in a touring caravan. The family would pack up the car and caravan with every necessity. Hitching up the car and van, the family would leave in the early hours to avoid traffic. Driving through the Welsh countryside at approximately 4 am. Once there, the caravan would be unhitched on a selected plot and Neil and his mum would be unceremoniously left for six weeks whilst his father went back to Manchester to work.

Located on the Llŷn peninsula, the site is located on an old quarry that protrudes into Cardigan Bay. The harbour and marina are on one side and the open sea on the other. Neil's inheritance also meant we could buy a boat. As a child, Neil spent many hours on the water. His best friend had a small boat with an outboard engine, which was frequently seen bobbing around the bay for pleasure, fishing or annoying the harbour master by breaking the strict four knots speed limit in the harbour. Our first investment was a small yellow and white Maxum boat (the model, horsepower and engine size meant nothing to me however the thought of speeding across the open sea chasing dolphins and seals is very appealing). We then had the opportunity to upgrade to a larger Chaparral model. After much deliberation, we named her 'Murfran's Spirit' after Neil's parents, Muriel and Frank. She now sits on her trailer in the park and launch facility of Bluewater Marina, waiting for calm waters and sunny skies.

We drive down after I finish work on Maundy Thursday. Avoiding the drive along the A55 (and the probable Easter car prangs and traffic jams), we drive across to Bala and through to Porthmadog. We have the essential groceries in the boot of the car, namely sausages, bacon, eggs, bread, milk and alcohol (no wonder I get strange looks in Asda). In hindsight, we could stop at the Tesco in Porthmadog or Asda in Pwllheli on arrival but my routine is what it is!!! If nothing else, we are sure to have a fun evening and a filling breakfast.

Moe and Graham join us later and we spend the evening in the on-site club where a Jersey boys' tribute band, the Jersey Notes are playing. Prosecco, beers, music and great friends. What more could I want? Saturday, we drive out to Porthmadog. We watch the steam trains build up momentum before taking expectant passengers and overexcited children out towards the slate mines and castles that are scattered across the Welsh landscape. We have a Mexican meal booked at a local restaurant for that evening (with the customary cocktails). The Pontoon Restaurant (named such as it is located next to the pontoon in the harbour) is within walking distance of the site and was originally the power boat club 'back in the day' (my husband informs me). The empty building opened as a 'popup bar' set up for one summer season a couple of years ago and hasn't closed since, with bookings having to be made months in advance due to its popularity. Sunday lunch is also already pre-booked. I'm so glad nobody thought to bring Easter eggs (note to self: still need to lose weight). After lunch, we drive out to Portmeirion. For anyone that hasn't been, it is a mock Italian village on the coast and it is beautiful with quaint shops and exceptional ice-cream. The sun is out and I don't have a care in the world.

The following morning is completely different. I cannot explain why but I am upset. I can't say what has triggered this outburst. Why this morning? Why now? Everyone else is up. The kettle is on, so I put on my dressing gown and walk into the lounge and the only sentence spoken is "Good morning, How are you?" No sooner has this simple question been asked than the tears start. I turn back into the bedroom. Neil follows. I want to be angry over such a stupid question "How am I?" How do you think I am? But I'm not angry. I don't know what I am!!! Nothing more can be said. I shower and dress and start the day again.

I have my sanctuary by the sea, I have my friends and I have my life.

Holiday Stress –
Merry Month of May!

Wednesday, 8 May

Two weeks after Easter and after the May Bank Holiday in Wales, we are back to reality and another appointment to attend. This morning we are back at the Nightingale Centre for my pre-operation meeting and I need to have a magseed implanted. This is a marker to help guide the surgeon to the affected area to remove it. It is 5 mm long…smaller than a grain of rice. At this point it will take some convincing that a potentially terminal disease can be located and eradicated through locating something less than one centimetre long.

The procedure is completed and I have progressed from my night-time dream status of being Lara Croft to being virtually the bionic woman! I have a titanium clip in my left breast, I just don't have any superpowers!

The next weekend we are back in Wales. I look out over Cardigan Bay wondering when and if we will return. I have that one last week at work to get everything in order; delegate work, update reports, delete emails, put on my 'out of office' automatic email response. This is a surreal experience. I don't know when I will return to this office or my desk.

Thursday, 16 May

Today is the start of our city break. Our hand-luggage is prepared. Our drag-a-bags, as I call them, are packed with every item of clothing to cater for every season and we are just under our weight allowances, which is a miracle in itself. We get a taxi to Manchester Airport and board our Easyjet flight to Pisa. I have sailed through airport security, smuggling through my little piece of metal. No alarms, no problems. My secret is safe with us.

We locate our hotel and set off to explore. We reach the university area on graduation day. The girls have their best dresses on and floral crowns, akin to the laurel wreathes worn by Roman emperors. We decide to stop here for a beer and watch these emotional moments where friends celebrate, and emotional parents compare their family achievements. The irony of us stopping at this little bar is that, after travelling from the UK, our lager is served in Joseph Holts' glasses!

The Leaning Tower is, of course, a must, with the obligatory 'hold up the tower' photograph. The following day, we get the train into Florence. The hotel is on one of the side-streets leading from the Duomo. A great location for the price we paid. We have the best time, sightseeing, walking miles in sunshine and showers, eating the most succulent Fiorentina steaks, drinking the best wines, cocktails in the Hard Rock café. Despite all this fun, I'm not sure if I've ever lit so many candles in so many churches as I do here, saying a prayer every time, whether the candle be lit by taper or a one euro payment in a slot where the flame bursts into life through the Italian electricity grid. This bloody disease is always in the back of my mind. We do a tour of the locations linked to the author Dan Browns book *Inferno*. The story is about an obsession in trying to control population numbers by releasing a deadly virus. It is linked to the real Dante's inferno. His depiction of a journey through nine circles of torment that is hell. We see a copy of Dante's death mask in the Uffizi Gallery. Now I have more questions. What is hell? Is my illness a virus? Why do so many people get some form of cancer? What would my death mask look like? Is there any point in wasting my time worrying? Probably not.

The sun is out and I'm in Italy with my husband. We wander over the famous Ponte Vecchio Bridge, lined with various shops, the jeweller's shops full of extravagant bling beyond our budget. We wander around the gorgeous Boboli Gardens to finish off our holiday. The time comes to fly home to the inevitable but now the plan unravels.

We return to Pisa International Airport. The thought of my operation the following day is lurking, but I know I can't change anything. Then we see the departure boards. FLIGHTS CANCELLED!!! Not just ours, nearly every flight. I feel my blood pressure rise and the tears start. We're not going home. The Italian airport staff are on strike. Now the emotional versus logical moments kick in. We're stranded in Italy. I have two pieces of hand luggage and emotional luggage to carry. I need to ring the hospital. I need to ring Moe who is taking us to the hospital and going on holiday the day after. How long are we stranded here for? For some bizarre reason, subconsciously wanting a friendly voice, I ring her first. I know she is at work and my voice starts wavering when she answers. I explain the facts as best I can through my trembling breaking voice. "We are stranded, I won't need your chauffeuring services to the hospital for my operation because I won't be there." She is off on her family holiday to

Tenerife before we will get home. I wish her a nice holiday and the dial tone tells me the call is over. I don't want to speak to the hospital on the phone from a foreign airport but have no choice. I explain the situation. The operation needs to be rearranged. A bizarre sequence of events.

I now have to contact Easyjet. Being a budget airline, they don't have airport representation. I now realise there is a one-hour time difference between Italy and the UK and the offices aren't open. An older couple next to us try to contact their travel agent. They are not as technologically 'savvy' as us so we try and assist them through my phone internet connection but to no avail. The lady is in tears as she rings their son for any assistance and comfort that can be offered.

Two hours later, our necessary arrangements are in place. The first available flight home is to Luton the following Friday so we now have three more days in Pisa. Accommodation is provided not far from the airport on full board basis, within walking distance of the city. Again, I know I can't change anything. Despite the circumstances, we make the most of this time seeing far more of the city; Roman aqueducts, fortifications and more bars and restaurants to sample.

Friday comes and we find ourselves back at the Pisa Airport. Flight secured, we arrive back in Luton and head straight to the National Express coach desk to be told that the next available coach to Manchester is at 7 pm with a one-hour stop in Birmingham. We would arrive in Manchester at 2 am. I have the strongest need to be at home in our own bed, but the thought of Manchester city centre at that time in the morning is not appealing at all. With the prospect of a 2-am-environment—the homeless on the streets, those unfortunates addicted to this new spice drug (literally zombies asleep on their feet) and the hardcore night clubbers laughing, shouting, fighting or tripping over their own feet—we decide to get a room at the Luton Airport Travelodge. The last time we were at Luton Airport was 30 years ago and we were flying out to Cairo for our honeymoon. This was when the actress Lorraine Chase was a national treasure and a regular on our television screens, promoting the joys of flight from Luton Airport. It had approximately five departure gates then!!! Our stroll to the hotel couldn't have been timed better as within half an hour of our arrival every room has been booked. The following day we get the coach for the five-hour trip home and upon arrival at Manchester city centre, we treat ourselves to a well-deserved pint in the local Wetherspoons.

We get home and on the doormat is the ominous white window envelope with the NHS postmark on the front. Another date has been arranged. The normality kicks in.

The Big Day

Wednesday, 29 May

I have woken early, well I'm not sure if I ever slept. It is the 'big day' when this nightmare will be over. My bag is packed and Neil and I leave the house, shutting the front door with a touch of finality. At some point today, I'm going to be medically put to sleep. I really want to see my front door again.

It is 8 am and I am back at the Nightingale Centre waiting to be injected with a dye to assist the surgeon with the procedure. We wait and we wait. The dye hasn't arrived from the Christie Foundation Trust. It is produced daily in line with the operations going ahead and is 'somewhere within the large Wythenshawe Hospital complex'. It has been delivered; they just have to find it. This isn't helping my state of mind but Neil, my husband and my rock, gives me that reassuring look that always makes things a little better.

Nearly three hours later, I'm on a side ward on Ward 16, the women's surgical ward. I am wearing my jeans and sweatshirt, waiting on my next instructions. Nothing seems amiss, then a nurse tells me to change into a surgical gown. Just me and my husband in an empty ward of eight beds. The anaesthetist arrives to confirm my name, date of birth, hospital number on my wristband and I have to tell them what my operation is and which breast will be operated on. It's a strange feeling of apprehension and nerves. I'm having a general anaesthetic; I can't control anything and I won't be conscious. Then my name is called! The nurse asks if I'm capable of walking to the theatre with them. Of course I am, I'm not disabled. I have been diagnosed with a mild inconvenience.

I leave Neil sitting next to an empty bed.

The vision of beauty that is me now swishes along a public corridor. I could be flashing my rather large posterior through my theatre gown to any medical and non-medical spectator I pass but I don't care. Today I'm also modelling the 'not so attractive' attire of non-matching surgical stockings and a pair of flip flops. Nothing colour co-ordinated but I wear this ensemble with pride. Then I reach the waiting room…and wait. My consultant appears around the corner in his full blues to say hello and tell me that everything will be fine. I'm reading an out-of-date magazine, well, looking at the pictures. I imagine I'm in a waiting room of a railway station, waiting for that train to come out of that tunnel, hoping I can get off the track.

Again the anaesthetist arrives to confirm my name, date of birth, hospital number on my wristband and I have to tell him what my operation is and which breast. I fall asleep.

The operation is done. I come round in the recovery room quite quickly, talking and reiterating, after being asked the same question again, that I am Ruth, my date of birth hasn't changed, and my left breast has been mutilated. Obviously this isn't how I respond to the questions but it is what I'd like to say. The one thing I remember is the medical calculation:

water + food + toilet break = home. I'm still propped up on the bed when I'm wheeled back to the ward where Neil is still sitting. The ward nurse arrives with my medication (rather promptly for a hospital I notice—the pharmacy must be quiet) I am given my instructions; *don't get the dressings wet, bathe don't shower and follow the exercise regime as instructed* (there is a reason I cancelled my gym membership…twice). I also have my injections to have daily to avoid DVT. I had DVT years ago. How can that still have an impact? Injections for a month!!! I am now a self-injecting, non-working person with a deformed, ugly, scarred breast. What has suddenly happened?

Happy Days

Thursday, 6 June

A week has now passed since the operation and I have followed my instructions with military precision. Get out of bed, inject, 2 cups of coffee, bathe, moisturise, and exercise. The exercises are not to the extremity of my previous gym membership. I stand in the bedroom waving and stretching the arm on the scarred side like a broken windmill or deformed snow angel lying on the bed.

Today we are back at the Nightingale Centre for me to attend a breast rehabilitation course. Another trip out for the husband who patiently sits outside in the waiting area as I join other six women who've been through various breast operations. We discuss exercises, pain, bra sizes. This is probably the most bizarre conversation I've had with complete strangers. Women I've never met before, all going through the same issues, but we laugh.

The frustration and boredom has begun to affect me. I would usually drive to Wales quite happily and even though Neil has offered to split the driving, the thought of the journey tires me. Unbeknown to me I have no need to be depressed. Yet again Moe and Graham step up to the mark. They have booked leave from work and offer to chauffeur us. The day after we are back in Wales, at our Sanctuary by the Sea. It is now a bit of a joke that they're assisting us to get a weekend break for themselves. If that were true (which it obviously isn't) we wouldn't have cared. They have been working on a data cabling contract and involved in working nights at the Christie Cancer Hospital in Didsbury...ooh the irony...

I love being in their company. The sun is out. The tide is calm. The boat is still on the bloody trailer and I can change nothing.

We chill, we eat, we drink and we laugh and all is well with the world.

Tuesday, 11 June

Two months and two days after my diagnosis, I have an appointment for my results. I've ticked the boxes, I've had all the tests, had implants and my operation so radiotherapy therapy department, here I come. Let's dot the 'I's and cross the 'T's. As Neil and I park at the Nightingale Centre, everything seems a little more positive. The journey there was smoother with less traffic. The sun is out and the external look of the centre seems less foreboding. There is a light at the end of that tunnel. No mental train thundering towards me today. I'm confident I've beaten the invader.

Neil and I are taken into the same consulting room. The consultant I see today is of Indian descent. This brings back the memory of me walking to the operating theatre in surgical wrap-around gown, dodgy stockings and flip flops looking like a Gandhi disciple with no dress sense. I'm not sure any exonerated holy man would have seen this as humorous unlike myself. He enters the room followed by my Macmillan nurse.

As they both sit down, I find myself staring at them for any tell-tale sign of my results; a frown, a smile, a hand gesture…but nothing. The consultant begins the chat. He refers to the historical facts of my case of which we are all fully aware and reminds me that it had been explained that if there was a risk of secondary cells that may cause a problem I may need a second operation. At this point, I feel a little irritated. I know all this so let's proceed with the next words being "I'm pleased to say…"

The next word I hear is "unfortunately". No, please God, not again!!! Well, sorry, this is me, I'm having a medical hiccup? This cannot be happening…can it? That afternoon my positivity leaves my not-so-skinny frame. They have found cells too close to the original cluster. They can potentially become cancerous. I need to come back in for a second operation. That mental train was heading out of that tunnel again, and I'm still on the track.

Yet again I have to pick myself and dust myself down. I see the look in Neil's eyes where the look of disappointment he feels for me is hidden with that glimmer of positivity in the smile he gives.

We leave the building knowing the white window envelope with the NHS blue stamp will drop through our door again.

That evening we are at the theatre with friends watching the musical, *The Book of Mormon*, a rude religious comedy musical. The tickets were pre-booked. Apart from the physical discomfort that I've been carrying for the last two weeks irritating me as I try to get a comfortable posture in the

36

theatre seats, I now have today's news to deal with. The show temporarily takes my mind off these distractions and I laugh but my overactive brain now has another query! What is religion? A belief in a Divine being? If there is a God, he's not doing much for me at the moment. Did all those candles lit and prayers said in Italy count for nothing?

Reality Again,
Let's Crack On

Monday, 17 June

I realise my pain threshold is failing me in the breast region so the phone call is made and I drag my stalwart of a husband back to the Nightingale Centre. God, I should have shares in this place. We people watch, my name is called. It's like I have volunteered for Groundhog Day. My breast is drained of excess fluid.

Issues of fluid continue to be the theme of the day as we also have the stress of having a new bathroom installed. The original was dated but functional and now I am not sure why I chose this particular moment of my life for this upheaval (obviously I haven't got enough going on). Am I being productive or is stress and boredom attacking the bank account? The suite is installed, a new ceiling is installed, lower than the other with modern LED ceiling lights (yes, the 60-watt bulb and lampshade has gone), the size and colour of floor and wall tiles are agreed (sods law they are out of stock half way through being fitted so now we now have a plumber on a mission—chasing tiles…and a final payment). At least we have facilities and my daily morning soak in the bath was only disrupted for one day. Neil had agreed this home improvement was a great idea...or is that expensive politeness. Another thought to keep me awake at night.

Tuesday, 2 July

It is the day of my second pre-op and I had been told this could be done by phone but I have the letter so off we go. I now wish my car is like KITT—the car in television's *Knight Rider*, or any other vehicle with automatic pilot. I am convinced I can see our repetitive tyre tread crossing the tramlines as we drive back to the hospital. On arrival, we play the usual cat-and-mouse game around the various car parks, otherwise known as the 'spot the space, get the space'. I wonder how much fuel I use in all these visits. Eventually we park and return to the dreaded Ward 16. I know deep down that there are other females in there going through far worse than me, but that is something else I can do nothing about. My appointment should have been done by phone. A wasted journey, the only consolation is that Neil treats me to lunch. Another sleepless night.

The Scalpel Returns

Wednesday, 10 July

Groundhog Day! The stunning clinical ensemble is back on. I've already been told that the surgeon will go in through the original scar and the aftermath could be more painful. Six weeks of discomfort, healing and dealing and I have to go through all this discomfort again. I don't know if I'm frustrated or annoyed. I'm frustrated because I don't understand why all this couldn't have been dug out, scraped through or whatever procedure they use the first time around. I'm angry that my body is putting me through this. Why did I get cancer?

Yet again, I'm the only one on the ward. Same procedure as last time, same questions; name, date of birth, wristband check, type of operation, which side. I leave Neil behind as I am again escorted along the same route as last time towards the entourage of masked medics who wait for my return. Walking the mile, walking the green mile!!!

Different anaesthetist, same procedure as last time, same questions; name, date of birth, wristband check, type of operation, which side. Again, I have no options, no choices. Keep breathing through the operation, recovery room, talk, drink, eat, go to the toilet and be chauffeured home.

This time I am a quieter passenger going home. I'm not the backseat driver trying to direct my husband from lane-to-lane or commenting on how far away from the kerb he is when he turns a corner. I'm tired and want this ordeal to stop. I do know that other men and women are facing far worse than me but, at this moment I don't care. This is about me and I hurt.

The Quiz

Saturday, 20 July

The landlord and lady of the local pub have decided to have a charity night for cancer research.

This is a fabulous idea for a most worthwhile cause but my current feelings contradict what I should feel. This has obviously been discussed and been arranged because of my predicament. It is a great cause but it shouldn't be held because of me (deep down I know it is). I want to believe it is a pub charity night that coincides with my problems. A majority of people know someone affected by cancer. My brain is in overdrive. It should be held because people throughout the world need these charities and need funding. The NHS are being stretched through lack of funding and pharmaceutical overheads on the cost of manufacturing medication. Here's a quiz question: If I was to ask approximately how many different cancers there are, what would people guess? There are over 200 different types of cancer!!! Now there's a potential tie break question to refocus the aim of the evening. My dearest husband listens to me rant on for the next half an hour until I stop for breath. He calmly asks if I'm going to compile and compere the quiz as asked. "It will keep me busy," he tells me. I start to trawl through newspapers and old supplements for obscure celebrities for a picture round. So many years have passed since I stood in the pub with a microphone in my hand on a Sunday night shouting out the quiz questions. I would have heated discussions with contestants who, apparently, were not 'on their phones using google for assistance' or occasionally making a fool of myself when that one extra pint got in the way of some articulation skills. We all muddled through. And we laughed.

This evening I wear my blue *Join the Christie against cancer* T-shirt. This is a complimentary T-shirt I was awarded (along with a medal) ten months earlier when I decided to fundraise for cancer research by doing a sponsored skydive.

After seeing an advertisement on Facebook to do such a thing, I paid the registration of £25. For some bizarre reason, as I am afraid of heights, I had committed myself to jumping from a plane. As many others had (for whatever their personal reasons), we had convinced ourselves that it was a great idea to join more strangers, be strapped to a stranger and jump out of a plane over Blackpool at 13,000 feet. Neil and I travelled up to Lancaster for an afternoon and evening out. Chauffeured again by our trusted mates (and witnesses to this event), I received 'the green light' text that evening and the following day found myself at the Black Knights Parachute Centre strapped to a stranger and jumping out of a plane hurtling towards earth. This is until the parachute opens, the wind rush stops and the silence and the views become the most peaceful place in the world. I raised £1600 through sponsorship on the back of that act of profitable stupidity. How things have changed in the last ten months. How I will need the Christie?

The charity evening begins steadily. A few of the locals are away and some have other commitments but there is a steady stream of customers at the bar, finding seats throughout the establishment. I'm hoping that is a good sign that they will be staying for at least a short while. I start the evening with my quiz, hopefully ensuring I retain customer's interest while we are all sober. After the twenty questions and picture round, I give the answers before splitting the proceeds between the charity and the winning team. The winning team also have a trophy presented. I'm not sure how the landlord got his hands on a trophy but it takes centre stage with me and the winning team in the photograph.

The son-in-law of the landlord and landlady has his head shaved and there is a game of bingo, a raffle and an auction. One of the regulars generously goes home and returns with a framed and signed Manchester United football shirt to be auctioned as it was 'gathering dust'. A comedian known as Tiny Tim and the DJ hosting the evening have given their time for free. Tiny Tim acts the part of a child 'aged 3 going on 6' and puts him in adult scenarios which is funny and some adults in the pub recognise these scenarios. The pub isn't very busy, but it is fun. We raise £800.

Results Day Again

Tuesday, 30 July

It is Tuesday and the day of my long-awaited hospital appointment for my results. The appointment is at 3 pm so I try to stay busy at home. There is actually nothing to do. All domestic chores have been done by Neil—Neil the househusband, Neil the nursemaid, Neil the cook.

It is ten weeks since I finished work for us to go on our Italian holiday. I have never been so bored or frustrated. Neil couldn't be more loving and protective but I have never been a person to be wrapped in cotton wool. I have tried to do bits around the house but despite his insistence in doing everything and my stubbornness in trying to do anything, we are still talking. Even though I am continuing with my exercises and cream application, I still feel my scars pull when I reach for a cupboard door or something at height. I assumed the healing would be a quick process but as Neil points out, there have been two operations, two incisions in the same place. I hope there won't be any more.

We arrive back at the Nightingale Centre slightly early for the appointment. The waiting game at home was getting the better of me and I have virtually dragged Neil through the front door listing every possible reason why we had to be there early, from traffic to staffing levels at the hospital.

Different faces sit around, waiting for their names to be called. All with different reasons for being there. Different fears, different expectations. I can't afford to have expectations, not after last time, just that same feeling in the pit of my stomach. Then my name is called. Here we are again, the same consultancy room as the previous times, and we sit and we wait.

The consultant enters the room followed by my Macmillan nurse. The same scenario as last time. Surely it can't be bad news again. He starts to explain what they did the second time around and check my scars. I'm not sure I'm taking in what he's telling me. I look at Neil hoping he understands what is being said. The one thing I do register is the fact that they have removed all cancerous cells. This announcement seems as surreal as being told I had breast cancer four months ago. I need three weeks radiotherapy and to take a tablet for the next five years to stem any further problems. I don't have to see any consultant again. He leaves the room. The nurse is now in his seat. "Have you any questions?" I think about that train, but now I'm on it. I'm the driver in control, standing on the footplate at the front, stoking the fire of a steam engine, racing out of that long tunnel, towards the sun, the countryside and my life. And I cry, properly, for the first time throughout this whole horrible process and I want to tell everyone, throw open the consultancy room door and tell the world.

As we leave, I walk past all the people sitting in the waiting area as I'd done in the past. I am bodily intact with a head full of hair. I see the bald lady—the scars of chemotherapy, the couples in tears and I pray for them. Perhaps there is a God, a Divine being to help them.

Happy Times

August

This month is the best I have felt for a while; no fears, no doubts and no evil cells potentially eating away at me.

The sun is out and we appear to be having a British summer. Neil, myself, Moe and Graham travel down to Woburn for the 2019 AIG Women's British Open Golf. We stay overnight and follow the golfers through to the final. The following day, we stop at Bletchley Park, the 19th-century mansion that became the principal centre of allied code-breaking during the Second World War. There is only four of us here that know my secret.

On getting home, Graham sends me a screenshot from the golf being shown on Sky Sports. There, in the middle of the screen, is the champion-in-waiting about to take her shot, supported by Neil and me in the background. OK, perhaps it's a good job my illness has been an 'open' secret, at least with work colleagues. I am on sick leave from work and blatantly on show on Sky Sports TV station.

Other things are on my mind. It still riles me that the boat hasn't touched the water this year (apart from with a bucket and sponge). The only consolation I have is that, between the weather and the company we have had, it just hasn't been possible. The decision has been taken out of my hands so I must put this to the back of my mind. Previous visits to the marina have ended in heated discussions with Neil because "I am well". Mr Sensibility of a husband points out that "it only takes an emergency or rogue wave to affect your scarring and internal stitches…and it's been weeks, not years since your operation." That's me told.

Later that month, I evict Neil from our 'Sanctuary by the Sea' in Wales and there is a girlie weekend away with Moe, her sister Janet and another friend Theresa, who is celebrating her birthday. Not only have I evicted him. I have also left him without any mode of transport as I drive off with the three girls as if we are in a four-person version of Thelma and Louise, just managing to see through the rear-view mirror due to the excess baggage. We are only there for two nights!!! On arrival, the car is unloaded and a decision is made, I'm not sure by who, to go for a 'couple of drinks' in the on-site club. It quickly becomes apparent that the domestic skills such as cooking, unpacking, etc. that should shine through four women will not become apparent any time soon. The only activities this evening consist of raising glasses, returning to the van, changing into nightwear and raising more glasses.

The day after the liquid diet, an executive decision is made that solid intake (generally referred to as 'stodge') is the required breakfast so off to Wetherspoons we go—all feeling remarkably well.

It is a birthday weekend. We drink, we eat, we go to Portmeirion and we go crabbing off the jetty. Four females that could be classed as middle-aged, with crabbing lines, smoked bacon bait and buckets. This may be considered a trivial activity in the guide and scout community however the competitive streak, along with the fear of crabs scurrying around the jetty after some members of the group, leads to some merriment.

The following weekend, August Bank Holiday, is the husband's 60th. We've been generously given the chalet next door (rent-free) for our neighbours and friends from home. Graham and Moe are staying with us, whilst Paul and Sandra and Fran and Anne move into this weekend accommodation. The men have arranged a round of golf at Pwllheli Golf Club so the ladies decorate the club and we surprise Neil on his return with a cake, cards and gifts and some of the friends we've made on-site also come in. We all have a fab meal in the Whitehall pub in town on the Saturday evening, followed by cocktails.

Sunday is a lazy day. The day of the site talent show dawns, the sun is out. Some of us drift in and out of town. Some of us drift in and out of sleep. Neil and I drift in and out of Weatherspoon, where we all return for tea. Forgetting it is Bank Holiday, we find ourselves stranded in town. There, by the grace of God, is one taxi and the site manager chauffeuring us back to the club.

Nearly the Last Hurdle

Friday, 30 August

Today we attend the Christie Centre Salford Royal for my scan plan and tattoos. Well, it's a change of scenery from the Nightingale Centre. Something tells me the body art isn't going to be anything to show off in any non-designer swimwear I currently own. I meet the consultant to confirm my understanding of the procedure. Of course, I understand the procedure!!! Well, being truthful, perhaps I should have looked into it a bit more, but I've read so much and googled so much, I've confused myself with the rights and wrongs of my problems.

I sit in the waiting room with Neil and wait. And then my name is called.

I change into a designer Velcro top, emblazoned with *The Christie* logo. In fact, it is a top of different pieces held together by Velcro, ideal for a Velcro-obsessed stripper who wants to remove any sleeve, side panel or any bit of material to flash a bit of anatomy.

I'm taken into the radiology room to see a CT scanner tube that looks like a bizarre polo mint and what appears to be the most uncomfortable bed I've ever seen.

I lie down, put my feet up against the footboard, a metal mound is at the base of my back, my head is positioned on a head rest and my hands are put on rests above my head. No handcuffs? I need to let that fetish thought go! Everything of my position is measured. The angles of my whole posture are logged, computed to ensure it is the same for every appointment. I'm shunted in and out of the tube to ensure the lasers align. I am now the train in that tunnel. The grand tattoo is actually three dots made by a radiographer with a marker pen (No high tech, multi-coloured design).

I get dressed and leave the building with my treatment itinerary, my shirt hiding my new tattoos and felt tip artwork and carrying the new Velcro blouse that is mine to take home. Not sure I'll be buying a matching handbag anytime soon!!! My secret is safe with us.

We pack up the car and head off to our Sanctuary by the Sea, to be followed by Moe and Graham. Those darn pesky kids are back!!! But who could ask for better mates who change their plans to be with us? On Saturday, after the customary sausage sandwiches and showers, we drive to Porthmadog. Even my shower has to include a plan; don't scrub the pen tattoos. Problem being, the other pen marks that have been drawn on me, dot here, arrow there, don't want to come off either (note to self: contact NHS stationery department regarding indelible markers).

After a wander to the steam railway, around the shops and a stop for liquid refreshment, we drive back to Criccieth, where a building called the Spice Bank attracts our attention. The bank now serves Korma, not currency so that is our dining planned. Another great weekend of dance and copious amounts of alcohol.

Bone Scan

Another day, another appointment. We are back at the Nightingale Centre at Wythenshawe Hospital as I need a bone scan. The density of the calcium in my bones needs to be checked as the medication I am on for the next five years can cause side-effects such as osteoporosis. Something else for me to worry about. I'm called in for my appointment, leaving poor Neil on his own in the waiting room, waiting for me…again. Now I'm on a bed, in my underwear, in various poses that will never make it to *Playboy* or *Vogue* while a laser scans my hips, pelvis and spine. It is more abnormality in my life. Put your legs on the box, from the knees. 50 shades of…Shit, these people love me more on the inside than the outside. Perhaps externally I'm less interesting. Even though I now hate attending this place because of what it represents, there is that something in the name 'The Nightingale Centre'. Florence Nightingale made her name as the most outstanding nurse in the Crimean War and the song *A Nightingale sang in Berkeley Square*. The smallest things keep my brain active.

The Final Chapter

Friday, 6 September

Today is my brother's 46th birthday. This isn't a 'big' birthday in the grand scheme of things and his card should be dropping through the letter box at some time that morning, but my deed is done. I'm not sure why this is significant apart from the date. I'm not even sure he knows how I am celebrating his birthday. Strangely, today feels like it is the start of part two of my experiences this year. A second chapter in the story of me. The operations are done, the meetings have been held, the diagnosis explained and dealt with. The cancer removed. Wythenshawe Hospital and the Nightingale Centre are a memory and the Christie Unit and Salford Royal is the future.

Today I am attending my first appointment for radiotherapy at The Christie Unit at Salford Royal. We get there at 2:15 pm—half an hour early. I would say this is because I need to be mentally prepared and I hope I get in early. The actual reason is far more domesticated. We think shopping for a new rug for the caravan will take my mind of today's events. Mission fail. No purchase and now I have given myself another extra half an hour to sit around and stress. We sit in the waiting area. I flick through the old *Take A Break* magazines, doing crosswords and word searches that others have got tired of, completing those that are incomplete due to the interruption of an appointment or a lack of brain cells they were born with to work it out!!!

Today is a very busy day. Just my luck for turning up early. There is a two-hour delay so we sit drinking coffee and people-watch. My stress level fluctuates like a bottle in my beloved Cardigan Bay, somewhere between a sandy beach and rocky outcrop, bobbing about not getting very far. Finally, my name is called. Two nurses take me to a side room to explain the procedure. They discuss what I have been through previously, what these radiotherapy sessions consist of and any possible side-effects. I haven't considered any side-effects. I assumed, in a basic way that it would be a daily 'zap and go'. I realise there may be more to this than meets the eye.

I return to the waiting area and re-join Neil where I repeat exactly what I have been told, including the possible side-effects. As he correctly points out that this is the last phase, the last episode of this dramatic series. As the Joker asked in the *Batman* film, "you ever dance with the devil in the pale moonlight?" I have but now I'm about to leave the dance floor.

My name is called. I put on my designer Velcro ensemble and enter the treatment room.

The machine is not a CT scanner. It is a mobile arm that moves over me. My permanent tattoos are intact, my measurements are confirmed by the radiologist with their pens and rulers. I am now lying there like a bull's eye. Even the radiotherapists leave the room. I am now alone. The crosshairs of a green laser pinpoint my breast. I can only think of James Bond in the film *Goldfinger* in the scene when he is tied to a bed with a laser on him. Then those immortal words "No, Mr Bond, I expect you to die." The laser moves from one side of my breast to the other, infiltrating the areas identified, yet I feel nothing. No sooner has the process begun than it is complete. The treatment is over. Three hours later, my first box is ticked.

Monday, 9 September

Today is our 30th wedding anniversary. We are not where I thought we would be. My plan was a weekend in Budapest and on this day, we would be having a romantic river cruise on the Danube with a meal and a nice bottle of wine. Instead it is 7:00 am and the most I can look forward to is a couple of slices of toast near the Bridgewater Canal. Neil and I leave the house. My bag is packed, not with the shorts, toiletries and suntan lotion we had discussed previously but my daily schedule and designer Velcro blouse for my appointment. This was definitely not my plan for today. Damned cancer. I confirm name, address and date of birth. My body is penned and measured, and the procedure starts. As I lie there alone, I notice six of the ceiling tiles are photos that form a view of the sky through autumn leaves. I am lying in this forest. For those minutes we are on that holiday and my eyes fill with tears. Then the radiologists enter the room, and reality resumes. I now have a meeting with the physiotherapist and as we wait, a lady rings the bell. That one sound that tells you that someone is now in remission, treatments are over and they can get back to normality. And my eyes fill with tears.

There is my goal, hanging on the wall.

I am done here for the day. We go out for lunch to Altrincham Golf Course. No sun or sea. Plans are on hold. My world is 8 am appointments every day, Monday to Friday for three weeks. This is now my life.

Appointments

I decide that I can attend these appointments on my own. Nobody else can do anything for me or make the situation change or go away, not even Neil. He has offered but dragging him from the 13.5 tog duvet to sit around is a pointless exercise. The medical team have confirmed that my driving will not be impaired with the treatment and I count my blessings that my appointments have been made for 8 am so I'm not waiting around at home, arguing with the househusband over household chores.

As I drive through the barrier, I seem to have a regular parking space now. My little Mazda nestles in between two large saloon cars as if it's being protected. The same cars that are there every morning. It seems strange sitting in this large waiting area on my own. Two gentlemen sit in the same area, I assume they are the other cars' owners. It is the first week and as the appointments continue and the days pass, a sense of familiarity starts to kick in. I am no longer that lonely woman waiting for the radiologists to call me at an unearthly hour in the morning (8 am has been an ungodly hour since I finished work in May).

Within the first week, I am on first-name terms with the receptionist and the two gentlemen I share my mornings with.

"Good mornings" start the day with the receptionists, the radiologists, the fellow patients. Acknowledgements and smiles, a nod of the head, a hello is now the norm. The three musketeers of radiotherapy (as we call ourselves) discuss every subject from our plans for the day to the side-effects of the treatments but it is always the daily routine, confirm personal details, confirm measurements with pen and ruler, have treatment and leave. That is now normality. I'm a human dot-to-dot. Everyone is on the same side, fighting the same battle. I have new breakfast buddies, the prostate pals. We are the three musketeers fighting the big 'C'.

Driving home every morning, I notice the same groups of schoolchildren walking and cycling to another stressful day of education. The same workmen calling in the bakery. Their lives go on and the world turns.

The one thing I have to do is to keep a sense of normality; go shopping, get out walking and go to the pub. I have theatre trips. I go to see Dolly Parton musical 9-5, a fab musical based around an office. I remember a 7 am to 4 pm work day. Oh, to get back there.

Thursday, 19 September

The weather is sunny so we have a day out on the East Lancashire Railway. It is a gift for my husband's 60th. A steam train from Bury to Rawtenstall. But first I have my treatment. I feel tired and my fatigued brain is working overtime today. Every morning I drive to the Christie car park at Salford Royal Hospital. Today I realise I drive past the mortuary. This isn't really significant, but today, to me, it is. I don't know why. Perhaps because we're going on a train. I'm going on a train.

That train that is in my head, my mental journey is now real. I am on a platform, I am in a carriage being pulled by a steam locomotive, looking out at green fields and into steam filled tunnels, and racing out of that long tunnel towards the sun, the countryside and my life. I am OK.

Thursday, 26 September – THE END

Today is the day. Neil and I are at the Salford Royal Christie Unit. My last treatment. The breakfast crew are with me. The three musketeers are all together. My new friends. We have agreed that I will ring the bell when they have had their treatments. I wait for them, not to brag that my treatment is done, but to give them hope and positivity for their future. I ring the bell. The crew gives me a congratulations card and we hug and say goodbye. I walk through those sliding doors one last time. My battle is done. My invisible armour has gone. Now I can pull myself together. Normality will resume.

Emotional Surprise

I should feel the happiest buzz, the ecstasy of no more cancer, no more treatment. Strangely, there is a void. I have nothing to fight against. I feel emotionally drained. I'm sitting on that railway station platform on my own. The tracks are empty and it's silent. The train has left without me and there is an empty tunnel. I turn to the exit sign, through the turnstile, and onto the path that is the rest of my life with my husband, my best friends, my supporters and I know that the memory of the last six months will fade along with the scars. I had breast cancer and I have rung the bell, just like the train when it left the station.

I have no more appointments, yet the radiotherapy continues working inside me, from the inside out. I have the intermittent pain and heat sensations, the rash, and the itchiness. I have my lotions. I continue my exercises. The emotional side to this is different than before. I'm frustrated. I'm angry. I'm tired (fatigued is the medical term) and I get upset over the most stupid things. I am cured. I did attend that appointment. The NHS did save my life and my body still works and fights. Ringing the bell isn't the end of the journey everyone believes. It's no longer a train leaving a station, it's a boxing match. Every day is a round and a bell now rings at the end of every day. I am battered and bruised but I'm here and normality will resume. It's all a matter of time.

The Future – Holidays!

I return to work. It is as if the past months are a blur. Did it all happen? Normality has now resumed and holidays are coming, as the Coca Cola truck advert on the television constantly reminds us. More importantly we have holidays coming. We own an apartment in Tenerife for one week every year (rather like a timeshare but we never swap the weeks or location). We fly there with Graham and Moe for a week in the sun before Christmas…and we have a 'big' holiday to look forward to.

It's the 31 January, 2020 and our long awaited 'big' holiday has arrived. Twelve months previously we decided the husband's 60th birthday should be celebrated with a big holiday. Any excuse, but where to go. The Far East is one of the locations that has always been a possibility and at this point it becomes a reality. Neil, me, Moe and Graham stroll into the TUI store in the Trafford centre and book the Colours of the Far East Marella cruise.

So here we are, sitting at Manchester Airport waiting to board our Thomson Dreamliner 787 flight to Langkawi, Malaysia. The flight is 11 hours with eight hours' time difference so after various meals, drinks, films and the addictive *Jewel Game* (and minimal sleep), we arrive.

Wow!!! After everything that has happened, we are in the Far East. We land at Langkawi Airport, luggage intact, and board the Marella Discovery cruise ship.

After such a long flight, we head up to deck 10, quickly identified as a deck with the best view of our new location, and order four small bottles of beer as we wait for our luggage to be delivered to our cabins. The intensity of the sun's heat hits us immediately, ironically as we discuss the fact that one couple has a piece of hand-luggage each yet due to the restriction on size of liquid bottles that can be carried, all suntan lotion is in the suitcases. We order four more drinks whilst working our way through the packets of ultra-soft tissues and wet wipes in a bid to cool down. We make our way down to deck 6 where our cases stand in the corridor, various outfits struggling to get out and be placed in wardrobes and drawers in our new homes for two weeks. Task completed and we have all changed. Holiday clothing of vest tops, shorts and flip flops become the attire of the day. We set off to explore the ship. For a vessel catering approximately 1600 guests, we all get our sense of direction relatively quickly.

The Central Atrium is what we call our 'muster point'. This is the actual name given to the point where every passenger must gather, when instructed, in their own designated points for the lifeboat drill (a cruising necessity). For the four of us, our muster station (the atrium) is our meeting point for trips ashore, drinks before changing for dinner, drinks after changing for dinner and overall central meeting point should we lose each other on board.

Our first destination is Penang, Malaysia. We walk into the city into an area called Little India. It is 33 degrees, but we are prepared. We have our Malaysian Ringgit currency, wet wipes, bottle of water and damp flannel. I have a strong feeling this is going to be the daily anti-dehydration pack in my knapsack. This place is an experience. Renowned for its street art, it has various street food which includes biryani on banana leaf that we share. This is eaten standing on the pavement where, upon completion, a builder working on an adjacent building offers his hosepipe, not to wash down the pavement of our spilt lunch but to wash our hands. The friendliness of the Malaysian people has certainly impressed so far.

We return to the ship and set sail into new adventures. On board that evening it is the 'dress to impress' evening where all passengers have the opportunity to meet the ship's captain and the head of departments. The men wear their dinner suits and the ladies wear their lovely dresses that only see the light of day on a very special occasion or this night on a cruise. My dress is a slightly bejewelled black three-quarter length strappy number. The picking of this frock has been quite a distressing experience. The scar where my biopsy was done in my armpit is healing well but I am still aware of it. Every dress in my wardrobe that could be appropriate for this holiday has been tried on prior to packing, for comfort, underwear issues (mainly bra comfort, restraints, padding, straps, strapless, wired or not…only the females will ever understand these problems). This was not an arduous task as the number of dresses I have is minimal and those that know me know I am a jeans and jumper girl. With the knowledge that, unless I'm going to be raving and waving my arms in the air like a deranged ape from which we are descendants, no passenger will be any the wiser so my secret still remains with me, my husband and our friends.

Kuala Lumpur is next on the itinerary and the band of four explorers head out from the port on foot, through the terminal towards the taxi rank. Those passengers going out on their organised excursions diligently queue to find out which bus or minibus they will be boarding. The taxi price is agreed upon and we all take our seats. It doesn't take long to realise our driver's knowledge of the spoken English language is minimal. Despite this, his understanding of the required sightseeing stops is the 'knowledge' of this Malaysian taxi driver. Our first stop is the Grand Palace. The taxi is parked, and we cross over a large central forecourt to the majestic gates. There are four guards on sentry duty. Two on foot, standing in the shade of the sentry boxes in their resplendent white uniforms and two on horseback. Although we know that some far eastern and oriental nationals wear face masks at home in Great Britain to reduce pollution intake and infection, it does seem strange to see military men doing the same but in a shade of pale blue that doesn't colour coordinate with any part of the uniform. We then visit the National War Memorial with an outstanding statue of troops in battle with the Malaysian flag flying proud. The inscription on it is dedicated to the heroic fighters in the cause of peace and freedom. The strange thing about this place is that for some reason a gentleman in a gold suit and trilby with a painted gold face posing in various obscure poses is here charging to have his photograph taken with tourists. The location of respect appears lost in the commercialisation of this.

The following day we dock at Singapore. The anti-dehydration knapsack is packed and the Singapore dollars are in the purse, along with my laminated currency exchange list I have for every destination. Our intrepid (previously a world backpacker for a year) friend Moe takes the lead with the map and following in her footsteps, we delve into the depths of the Singapore underground system. The colour routes and efficiency of running times embarrasses the British transport system. Not a surprise. We blow our budgets on ½ pints of lagers in the prestigious Raffles Hotel.

After a relaxing day at sea, we have sailed into the Gulf of Thailand and to the island of Koh Samui. It is a paradise island. A jewel in the Thailand crown. We are tendered ashore and soon strike a deal with a local taxi driver to show us the highlights of the island. We visit a picturesque waterfall where the view is blighted by the local elephants, tethered in chains, waiting to take unsuspecting or uncaring tourists on a trek. Temples and Buddha statues are scattered across the landscape and the sun shines down on the most turquoise of seas. We stop at the Fisherman's Village and enjoy a beer overlooking the golden sand with scattered large bean bags for sunbathers to rest on and look across the bay to the island of Ko Pha Ngan. It is at this point that Moe, yes the worldly wise back packer (though it was about 20 years ago), tells us that the island on the horizon is famous for the regular full moon parties and she had actually visited the island we are currently on (Koh Samui) on her previous adventures. Apparently in error, as her and her travelling companion got off the ferry on the wrong island!!!

Good job this guided tour was more successful!!!

The next few days we are off to mainland Thailand. We drop anchor in Laem Chabang, a two-hour drive from Bangkok. We decided to book an organised excursion on the ship to go to Bangkok and stay overnight. It is an interesting trip viewing temples and the Royal palace with lunch included but as Graham said—by the end of the day he was Buddha'd out. No more BUDDHA today!!! We have a gorgeous evening boat trip to see the buildings, bridges and temples lit up. Yes, alongside the sitting, standing and reclining Buddhas we saw earlier on in the day, we now have illuminated Buddhas. Our accommodation for the night is the Sheraton. Luxurious but even with this luxury, on an organised tour you know the pitfall…yes…leaving at 06:45 am. We visit the Floating Market and it is only when we are on our way to the ship and we stop for lunch that my heart sinks. I have no purse. Our purse has been stolen. I get a sickness in the pit of my stomach and I start to cry. I scour the coach. It's not on the floor. Damn the two girls in the public toilets before we left. I paid for all four of us for our pre-travel ablutions because I had small change. I know I put the purse back in my bag.

For those few minutes, the laughter, fun and appreciation of this trip, my travelling companions and everything that comes with, it means nothing. I am annoyed with myself and angry as I would be but this time there is something more. An embarrassment. The feeling that everyone on the coach is looking at me and judging me…the stupid tourist. Perhaps I am being punished for something just as I thought I was being punished ten months earlier. Previous to my health problem, this would have not been such a big deal but my self-doubt and insecurities have been exacerbated since then.

It was as much that thought that made me realise how things could have been worse. I do have my health, my happiness, my friends and I am in the most amazing part of the world, whilst the scum of Thailand attempt to live off a soon-to-be cancelled credit card, £200 sterling and minimal local currency. Apparently, the Thai baht is the only currency locals can 'officially' spend; my pounds will probably mean that some dodgy money transaction with a dodgy mate will have to take place. We find humour in the statement 'worse things happen at sea' as we head back to the cruise ship.

Things can be so much worse

Next we dock at Sihanoukville in Cambodia and leave the boat to find out that this town is currently a building site. We hire a *tuk-tuk* and the driver takes us out to the beach and around the town centre. There is a casino on every street but not the hotel infrastructure to cater for customers. The roads are ripped up and the workforce slave away in the heat with pickaxes wearing head-to-foot uniforms and overalls...and flip flops. No health and safety regulations here. I'm not sure this development plan has been thought through, but I won't tell the Russians and Chinese investors that. It is a short excursion which is probably a good thing as the following day's organised excursion starts at 7 am.

We are in Vietnam and the sun hasn't risen much before us this morning. Today we are going underground in the Cu Chi Tunnels. After the coach driver expertly negotiated the roads of Ho Cho Minh city (still known as Saigon to the Vietnamese) through the thousands of mopeds swarming the streets, we stop at a craft centre where ceramics are being handmade by locals, some with visible disabilities. On entering the shop, it is the sign above the door that catches my attention, "Your purchase significantly contributes in helping

those who are handicapped and suffered Agent Orange."
Agent Orange was a defoliant chemical used by the US
military as part of its chemical warfare programme to remove
forest and vegetation protecting the Viet Cong—the
Vietnamese liberation army. These are the people that
protected themselves in the tunnels of Cu Chi. Their
deformities and disabilities put my scars into perspective.
They are nothing but scratches.

We Have Two Days at Sea

The final day we return to the dock in Langkawi. We are
on the deck and in the port where it all began. We arrange a
deal with a taxi driver who agrees to take us around the sites
and to the tallest cable car in the world. Firstly, his itinerary
takes us to the mangrove swamps. Here he pulls up and
suggests we stop here for an hour or two and that he will wait
for us. We look at each other bemused as to why he thinks we
would waste a minimum of an hour in a mangrove swamp
testing our horticultural knowledge on identifying rubber
plants and swamp lilies (of which we know neither). It is only
when we reach the ticket office when we realise that this is an
opportunity to be on a traditional Malaysian longboat
speeding through the mangrove swamps, seeing fish farms,
wild Malaysian eagles and an actual bat cave. We agree that
this is an opportunity not to be missed and we pay for two
hours. It is reminiscent of a James Bond chase scene. As
promised, our taxi driver has waited (for his fare as much as
our company) and proceeds to take us to the cable car (Sky
cab). Ascending to the summit of the Machinchang Mountain,
we are overlooking the Malacca Straits. We can see our ship

in one direction and the airport in the other. We can see panoramic views of the Langkawi islands and across towards the Southern Thailand. In the distant, we can see the tsunami barrier that reminds us of nature's force. The top station is 708 m above sea level. Not being the best at heights, I do know that my distance from the railings will mean my photos will probably have a barrier or railing in shot somewhere. I encourage Neil, with his professional camera to snap away to his heart's content. All credit to Moe and Graham who can also see the earth beneath them as they walk on the sky bridge with a partially glass walkway.

We descend on to terra firma and find the Langkawi 3D museum. We do wonder why we have to take our shoes off on entering. It is a museum with paintings and murals across the walls and floors where, through a camera lens, the wall and floor become one 3D art painting where an individual can stand and appear to be fighting dragons or climbing ladders. Neil and I sail through a fictitious Venice and he wields Thor's hammer as our friends crawl across caverns and leap across craters of illusion.

We leave this behind and enter back into the real world and our journey back to the ship for our last night on our floating hotel.

We fly home tomorrow. I feel we've been away for longer than two weeks and after all our adventures, I know I have nothing to fear when I get home.

Closure

When I returned to work, it was only two months to Christmas.

I'm not a big Christmas fan. Not having children, I find it over commercialised, so I do prefer New Year. I see in any New Year as I always do, with copious amounts of alcohol and like a child entering a sweet shop or an amusement park. Everything is bright and exciting, new opportunities, new places to see, new things to do. Celebrating the new year of 2019 was just the same. The one difference is I didn't know that entering that amusement park of opportunity on 1 January, 2019 would put me on a rollercoaster I couldn't get off.

That appointment at the Nightingale Centre on the 9th of April has changed my life. People will assume that because I have had breast cancer and have been told I am all clear that everything is back to normal. I know that is what people think. They will assume all the boxes are ticked and all my emotions and feelings will be stored away in a mental box and pushed away to the back of my memory bank to gather dust.

Although I had the best cancer I could have, cancer still exists. God willing, I will never see it again but I am medically in remission. No-one will say cured. I am on medication for the next five years. I take a pill every day to suppress any further cancer. I take vitamin/calcium tablets for the osteopenia I was diagnosed with through my bone scan. I may rattle but I am well. I will go back to the Nightingale Centre every year for a mammogram and will have scars for the rest of my life to remind me that I am a survivor.

The one thing I have learnt is that no-one should take life for granted and that having someone to talk to does make life easier.

Embrace the friendships you have…and talk.

Never be afraid to learn and share…and talk.

Life can be unpredictable but that is what life is, nothing is guaranteed…so talk.

Live your life to the best of your ability and be proud of what you have achieved.

I have been to some of the most amazing places across the globe since I married 30 years ago—from a pyramid in Egypt to a pyramid hotel in Vegas. I've dived into coral reefs and flown above the Northern lights. From the Taj Mahal to temples in Thailand and still have so many more things to do and places to see.

I'm blessed, I'm lucky and I am a breast cancer survivor.